QUICK AND EASY
LOW FAT
LOW CARB DIET
RECIPES FOR
SENIORS

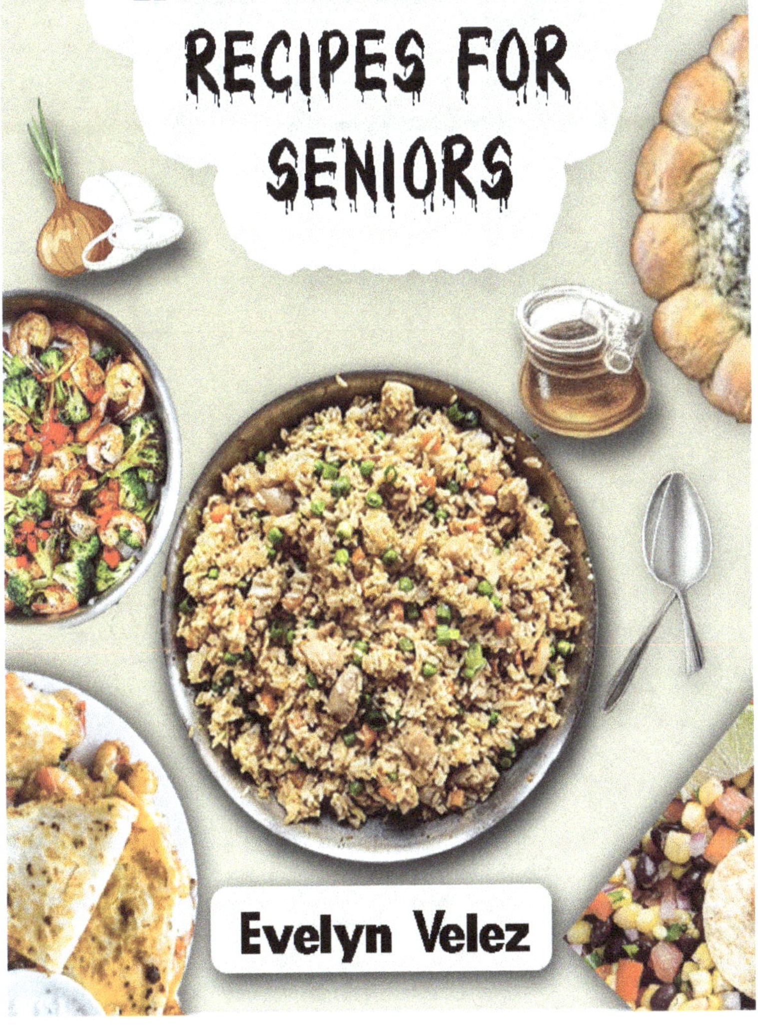

Evelyn Velez

Quick and Easy Low Fat Low Carb Diet Recipes For Seniors

Healthy Delicious Ideas For Breakfast, Lunch and Dinner With Original Photos

This ebook's content is exclusively intended for educational and informational purposes. The author does not diagnose or offer any medical advise because they are not medical professionals. Based on the author's own research and experience, the recipes and advice in this booklet are not meant to take the place of expert advice or consultation. The author disclaims all liability for any damages or losses that may result from using the advice in this booklet, and she does not guarantee any particular outcome. Before making any dietary or lifestyle changes, readers are urged to speak with their personal healthcare providers.

Introduction

Do you want to eat well-balanced meals without having to spend a lot of time and energy in the kitchen? Would you like to control your weight, blood pressure, blood sugar, and cholesterol by adopting a low-fat, low-carb diet? This book is for you if the answer to any of these questions is yes!

Many quick and simple low-fat, low-carb recipes that are especially geared toward a healthy lifestyle can be found in this ebook. You may readily get the basic, healthful, and reasonably priced ingredients used in these recipes at your neighborhood store. In addition, they offer ideas for serving, nutritional data, and methods for enhancing its flavor and texture.

This ebook contains recipes that will satisfy your cravings and nutritional requirements for breakfast, lunch, dinner, snacks, and desserts. You will learn how to cook:

- ➤ Spicy Grilled Calamari Salad
- ➤ Pot Shrimp and Broccoli
- ➤ Crispy Chipotle Shrimp Quesadilla
- ➤ Takeout-Level Chicken Fried Rice
- ➤ Artichoke Dip
- ➤ The Best Spinach Artichoke Dip
- ➤ Black Bean and Corn Relish

A low carb and low fat diet for seniors can have several benefits for their health and well-being. Some of the benefits are:

- As obesity is a risk factor for many chronic diseases, it can aid in weight loss and prevent obesity.

- It can enhance insulin sensitivity and lower blood sugar, which can help control or prevent diabetes.

- It can lower blood pressure and cholesterol, which helps lessen the chance of stroke and heart disease.

- It can supply enough fiber and protein to support bone health, muscle mass, and digestive health.

-It can provide a wide range of dishes and flavors, which can improve eating's pleasure and contentment.

A low-carb, low-fat diet for seniors, however, may also come with certain disadvantages, like:

- If the person has limited access to fresh and healthful foods, it could be challenging to follow and maintain.

- Consuming too much protein and insufficient water may raise the risk of osteoporosis, gout, and kidney stones.

- Insufficient brain glucose can have an impact on an individual's mood and cognitive abilities.

-Seniors' low-carb and low-fat diets should therefore be customized based on their needs, preferences, and health issues. In order to monitor the person's health and modify the diet as necessary, it should also be overseen by a physician or dietician.

Tips on how to avoid common pitfalls and challenges of a low carb and low fat diet:

-Hydrate yourself well. By burning fat for energy, your body loses water, which is why a low-carb, low-fat diet can make you dehydrated. Fatigue, headaches, constipation, and foul breath are more symptoms of dehydration. Drink two quarts of water or more each day to avoid this.

-Consume adequate fibre. Constipation can be avoided and blood sugar and cholesterol levels can be lowered by consuming fiber, which is beneficial to digestive health. You can better regulate your appetite and calorie consumption when you feel full and content after consuming fiber.
-Eat plenty of high-fiber, low-carb vegetables like celery, lettuce, spinach, and broccoli to ensure you receive adequate fiber. Add-ons such as chia seeds, flax seeds, and psyllium husk are

available.Make wise protein and fat choices. There are differences between all fats and proteins. A higher risk of heart disease and stroke is associated with certain lipids, including trans and saturated fats. There are certain proteins that can raise your risk of kidney problems and cancer, like red meat and processed meat. Choose low-fat dairy, avocado, almonds, seeds, fish, eggs, poultry, and olive oil as healthy fats and proteins to reduce your risk of these illnesses. The vital amino acids, fatty acids, vitamins, and minerals your body requires can be found in these foods.

-Take care of your nutrient balance. Diets low in fat and carbohydrates can lead to nutrient shortages, particularly if they are not balanced and diverse meals. Iron, B vitamins, calcium, and vitamin D are a few nutrients you could need to enhance or supplement. Your immune system, energy metabolism, blood formation, and bone health all depend on these nutrients. Eat items like leafy greens, mushrooms, tofu, beans, lentils, and fortified cereals to obtain these nutrients. To find out more about taking a multivitamin or a particular supplement, speak with your physician or dietician.

-Take note of your health. Individual differences in age, health, exercise level, and goals can all affect the impact of a low-carb and low-fat diet. Reduced inflammation, better blood sugar regulation, and quick weight loss are possible for certain persons. Some might suffer from exhaustion, fluctuations in mood, loss of muscle, and hormone abnormalities.

-Check your weight, blood pressure, blood sugar, cholesterol, and ketone levels on a regular basis to prevent any negative effects from occurring.

 To modify your diet to suit your needs and preferences, you can also consult a doctor or dietician.

If planned and followed carefully, a low-carbohydrate, low-fat diet can be an effective strategy for weight loss and improving health. You can get the benefits of a low-carb, low-fat diet by heeding these suggestions and avoiding the typical traps and difficulties therein.

Table of Content

Chicken Burger with Sun-Dried Tomato Aioli

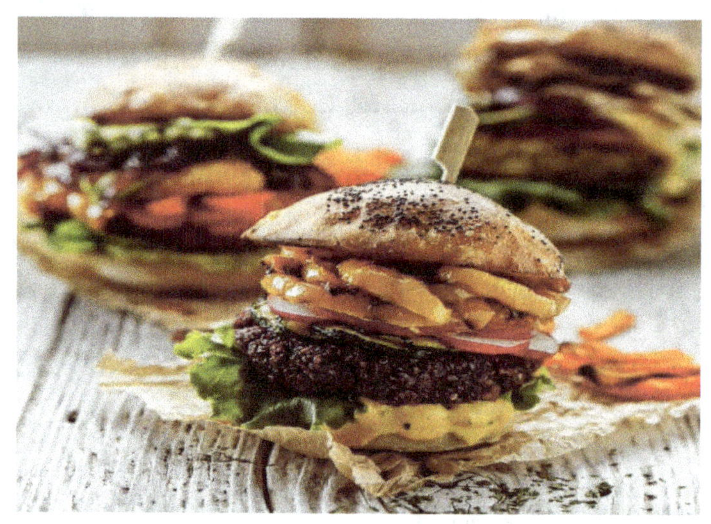

Ingredients

- ➢ 2 Tbsp olive oil mayonnaise
- ➢ 2 Tbsp chopped sun-dried tomatoes
- ➢ Juice of 1⁄2 lemon
- ➢ 2 cloves garlic, finely minced

- ➢ 1 tsp chopped fresh rosemary
- ➢ Salt and black pepper
- ➢ 1 lb lean ground chicken
- ➢ 4 whole-wheat or potato buns (or even English muffins), split
- ➢ 2 cups arugula, baby spinach, or mixed greens

Preparation

1. Combine the mayonnaise, lemon juice, sun-dried tomatoes, garlic, and rosemary in a mixing bowl. Add a dash of black pepper and salt for seasoning.
2. Preheat a grill, grill pan, or cast-iron skillet.
3. Gently mix the ground chicken with 1/2 teaspoon salt and 1/2 teaspoon black pepper.
4. Without overworking the meat, form the mixture into four patties until the chicken just comes together.
5. Add the burgers to the hot grill or skillet (if using a skillet, add a little oil).

6. Cook on the first side for 5 to 6
minutes, until a nice crust develops.
7. Flip and cook for an additional 3 to 4
minutes, until the burgers are firm but
ever so slightly yielding to the touch and
cooked through.
8. Remove the burgers.
9. Toast the buns while the grill or pan is
hot.
10. Layer the arugula on top of each
burger.
11. Crown with the bun tops

TIME

Time spent preparing: 20 minutes
- 10 minutes for cooking
- 30 minutes in total

RECIPE 2

Oatmeal Pancakes With Cinnamon Apples

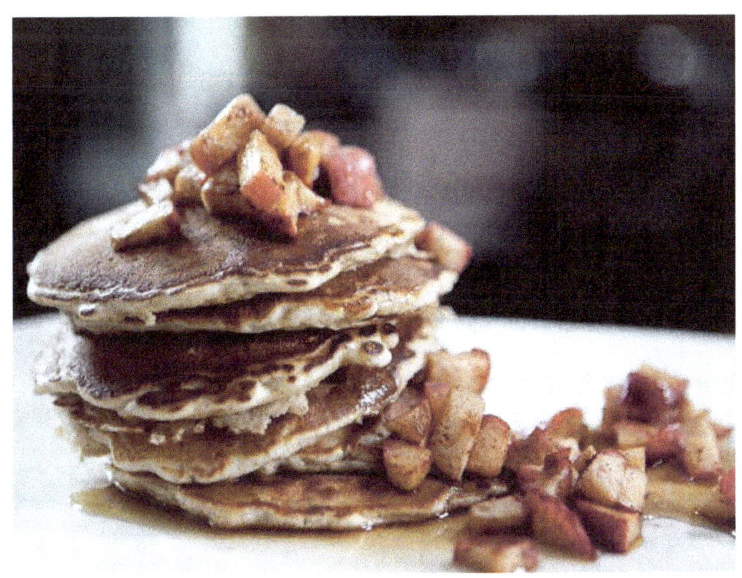

Ingredients

- ➢ 1 ½ cups buttermilk
- ➢ ¾ cup instant rolled oats
- ➢ ¾ cup whole wheat flour
- ➢ 2 Tbsp milk

- ➤ 1 Tbsp melted butter
- ➤ 1 ½ tsp baking powder
- ➤ ½ tsp baking soda
- ➤ Pinch of cinnamon (plus 1⁄8 tsp for the apples)
- ➤ Pinch of nutmeg
- ➤ 1 Granny Smith apple, peeled, cored, and chopped
- ➤ ½ cup apple juice
- ➤ 2 Tbsp brown sugar
- ➤ Butter or cooking spray
- ➤ Confectioners sugar

Preparation

1. In a large mixing basin, whisk together the buttermilk, oats, flour, milk, butter, baking soda, baking powder, nutmeg, and a touch of cinnamon.
2. Put the apple, apple juice, brown sugar, and the remaining 1/8 teaspoon cinnamon in a small saucepan and bring to a boil. Stir to gently incorporate, then remove and let rest for a few minutes1.

3. Set the oven's temperature to 200°F. Cook until the apple is tender and the liquid has thickened. Heat a sizable nonstick or cast-iron skillet over medium heat.
4. Spoon 1/4 cup portions of batter into the skillet, spreading it out into thin, even circles with a spatula after each round.
5. Cook until small bubbles form in the top of the batter, 2 to 3 minutes, then flip and cook for an additional 2 minutes.
6. Keep the pancakes warm in the oven while you finish cooking.
7. Serve topped with the warm apples and confectioners sugar, if desired.

RECIPE 3

Spicy Grilled Calamari Salad

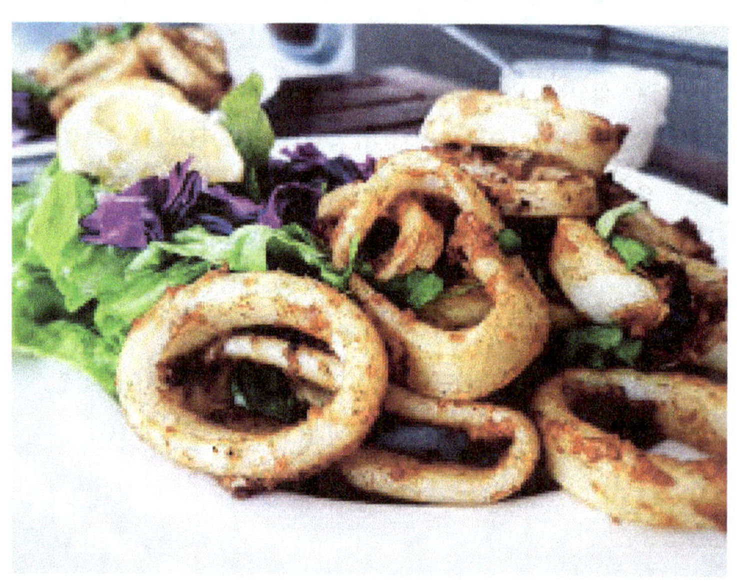

Ingredients

- ➤ 1 lb squid, cleaned, tentacles reserved for another use

- ➤ ½ Tbsp peanut or canola oil

- ➤ Salt and black pepper to taste

- ➢ Juice of 1 lime
- ➢ 1 Tbsp fish sauce
- ➢ 1 Tbsp sugar
- ➢ ½ Tbsp chili garlic sauce (preferably sambal oelek)
- ➢ 4 cups watercress (Watercress isn't always easy to find. Baby arugula, or even a few handfuls of basil leaves, can easily take its place here.)
- ➢ 1 small cucumber, peeled, seeded, and cut into matchsticks
- ➢ 1 medium tomato, chopped
- ➢ ½ red onion, very thinly sliced
- ➢ ¼ cup roasted peanuts

Preparation

1. Set the grill to preheat. Add plenty of black pepper and salt to the squid bodies after tossing them in the oil. The squid should be added to a very hot grill and cooked for about 5 minutes, or until it is lightly charred all over

2. Then, slice the grilled squid into ½" rings and combine the lime juice, fish

sauce, sugar, and chili sauce in a mixing
bowl and whisk to combine
3. Divide the salad among 4 plates. In a
salad bowl, toss the squid, watercress,
cucumber, tomato, onion, and peanuts
with the dressing[1].

RECIPE 4

Pot Shrimp and Broccoli

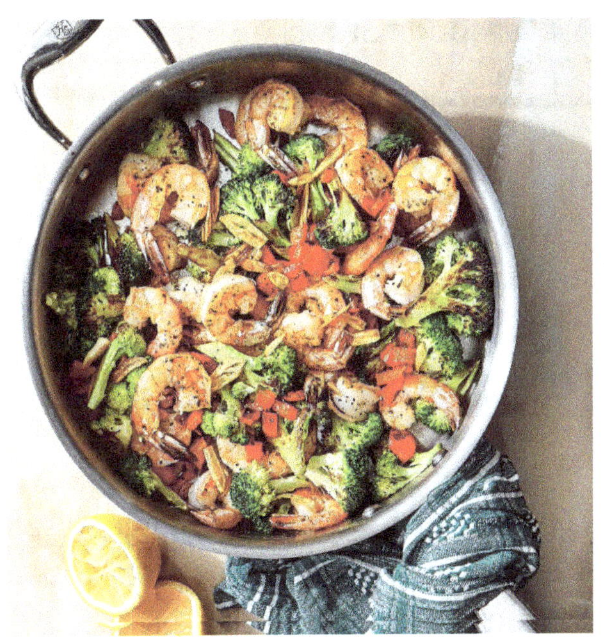

Ingredients

➢ 1 pound raw peeled and deveined shrimp

➢ 2 cups fresh broccoli florets

- ➢ ¼ cup reduced-sodium soy sauce
- ➢ 2 tablespoons oyster sauce
- ➢ 1 tablespoon rice vinegar
- ➢ 2 teaspoons sesame oil
- ➢ 1 teaspoon brown sugar
- ➢ 1 teaspoon Sriracha sauce
- ➢ 1 teaspoon minced garlic
- ➢ 2 tablespoons cornstarch
- ➢ 2 tablespoons cold water

Preparation

1. In a small bowl, whisk together soy sauce, oyster sauce, rice vinegar, sesame oil, brown sugar, Sriracha sauce, and garlic until smooth
2. Then, transfer the sauce to a multipurpose pressure cooker, like the Instant Pot.
3. Add shrimp.
4. Finally, cover and seal the cooker. Choose high pressure and set a 2 timer.

5. Let the pressure increase for ten minutes.
6. Meanwhile, whisk together the cornstarch and cold water until smooth.
7. Carefully release the pressure for approximately two minutes using the quick-release technique.
8. Let the cover open and take off.
9. Add the broccoli and cornstarch slurry.
10. Choose the Sauté option and cook for about two minutes, or until the sauce thickens and the broccoli is crisp-tender.

RECIPE 5

Crispy Chipotle Shrimp Quesadilla

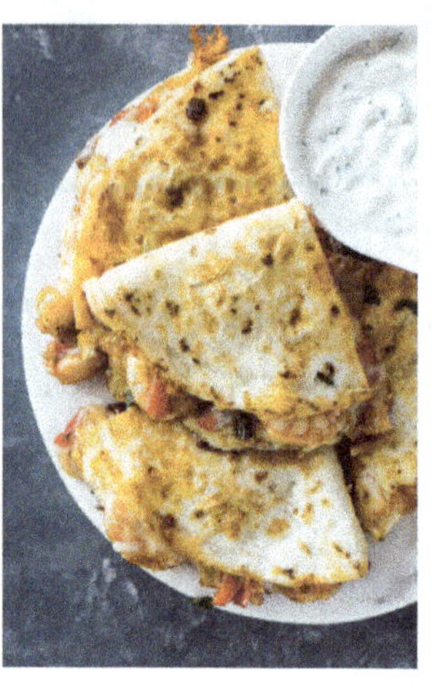

Ingredients

➢ 8 oz medium shrimp, peeled and deveined

➢ 1/2 cup orange juice

➢ 1 Tbsp canned chipotle pepper

➢ 2 cloves garlic, minced

➢ 1/2 Tbsp canola oil

➢ 1 medium onion, sliced

➢ 1 red or yellow bell pepper, sliced

➢ Salt and black pepper to taste

➢ 4 large whole-wheat tortillas

➢ 2 cups shredded Monterey Jack cheese

Preparation

1. Add the shrimp to the orange juice, chipotle pepper, and garlic mixture. Let the shrimp marinate for fifteen minutes.
2. Heat the oil in a large cast-iron skillet or sauté pan over medium-high heat.
3. Add the onion and pepper and cook for ten minutes, or until the outside is lightly charred.
4. Push the vegetables to the edges of the pan and place the shrimp in the center.
5. Season with salt and pepper to taste and sauté until cooked through, about 10 minutes.
6. Turn off the heat.
7. Spread cooking spray, oil, or butter on a different nonstick pan and heat it over medium-low heat.
8. Cook the quesadillas for about 5 minutes, or until the bottom is very crisp.

Then, turn them over and cook for an additional 2 to 3 minutes.

9. Cut the quesadillas into wedges and serve with salsa and some guacamole, if desired.

RECIPE 6

Takeout-Level Chicken Fried Rice

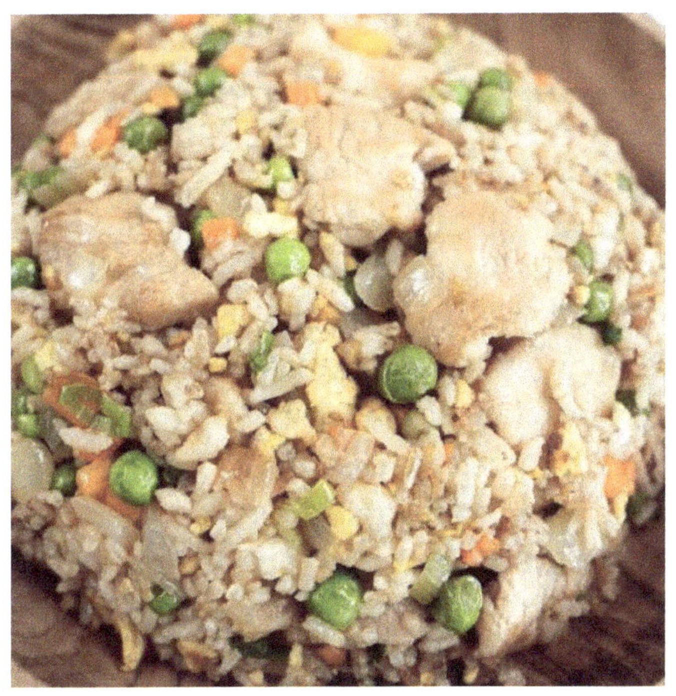

Ingredients

➢ Oil (both sesame and vegetable)

➢ Chicken breasts

➢ Frozen peas and carrots

➢ Green onions

➢ Garlic

➢ Eggs

➢ Cooked rice

➢ Low-sodium soy sauce

Preparation

1. Fill a big skillet with the oils and cubed chicken. Cook the chicken for about 5 minutes on medium-high heat, or until it's no longer pink inside.
2. Transfer the chicken to a platter and stir-fry the vegetables.
3. Add the peas, carrots, and green onions to the same skillet. After the garlic has softened, add it to the skillet.
4. Push the vegetables to one side and scramble the eggs on the other.
5. Return the chicken to the pan and then add the rice.
6. Drizzle everything with soy sauce and heat everything through.

RECIPE 7

Artichoke Dip

Simple Artichoke Dip

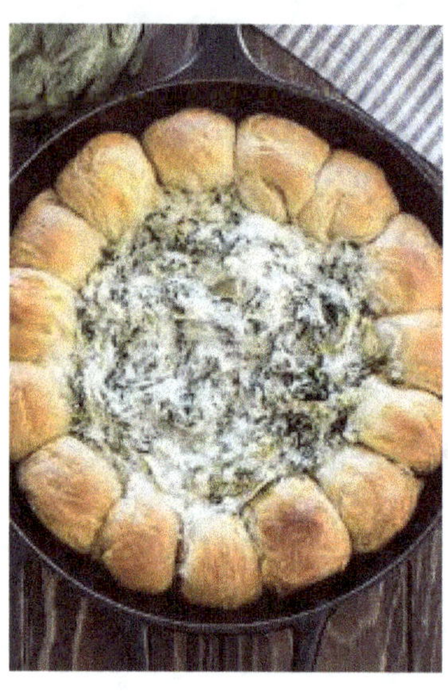

Ingredients

➢ 1 can (14 ounces) drained and chopped artichoke hearts, 1 cup grated Parmesan cheese, and 1 cup mayonnaise

Preparation

1. Turn the oven on to 375 degrees Fahrenheit (190 degrees Celsius).

2. Place artichoke hearts, mayonnaise, and Parmesan cheese in a bowl and stir until well incorporated.
3. Transfer mixture to a 9x13-inch baking dish.
4. Bake in a preheated oven for 15 to 20 minutes, or until bubbling and golden brown.

The Best Spinach Artichoke Dip

Ingredients

- Nonstick Cooking Spray, 8 ounces room temperature Cream Cheese, ½ cup Sour Cream, ¼ cup Mayonnaise, 1 grated garlic clove, 1 10-ounce box spinach (frozen leaf, thawed, drained, squeezed dry and coarsely chopped), 1 14-ounce can artichoke hearts (drained well and coarsely chopped), ½ cup shredded whole-milk mozzarella, ¾ cup freshly grated Parmesan cheese, Kosher salt (and

freshly ground black pepper),
Crackers (for serving).

Preparation

1. Stir to combine the artichokes,
mozzarella, and 1/2 cup of Parmesan
cheese.
2. Add pepper and salt for seasoning.
3. Spoon mixture into baking dish;
sprinkle remaining 1/4 cup Parmesan on
top.
4. Bake 20 to 25 minutes, or until dip
starts to bubble.

RECIPE 8

Black Bean and Corn Relish

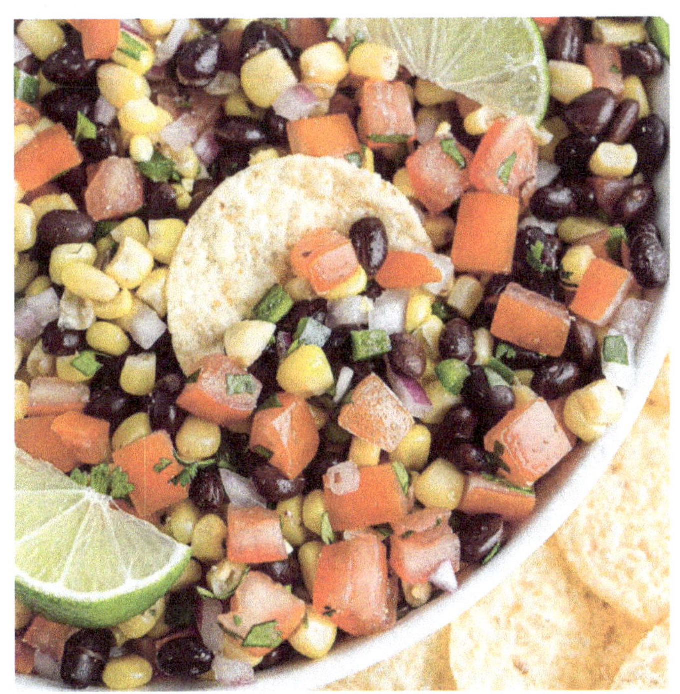

Ingredients

> ➢ 1 can (15.5 ounces) black beans,
> rinsed and drained (about 2 cups)

- ➢ 1 cup frozen corn kernels, thawed to room temperature
- ➢ 4 tomatoes, seeded and diced (about 3 cups)
- ➢ 2 garlic cloves, chopped
- ➢ 1/2 medium red onion, diced (about 1/2 cup)
- ➢ 1/2 cup chopped parsley
- ➢ 1 green, yellow or red bell pepper, seeded and diced (about 1 cup)
- ➢ 2 teaspoons sugar
- ➢ Juice from 1 lemon

Preparation

1. Combine all ingredients in a large basin.
2. Gently toss to incorporate.
3. Cover and chill for minimum 30 minutes to let flavors to meld.

RECIPE 9

Pan-fried Fish and Pan-fried Poultry

Pan-fried Fish

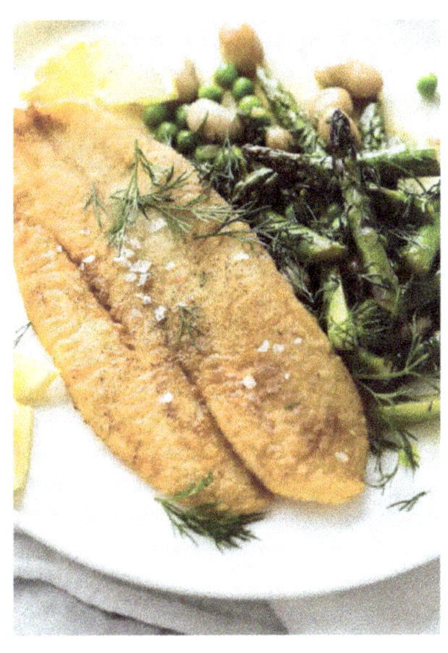

Ingredients

➢ Fish fillets, Flour, Bread crumbs, Seasoning, Eggs, Milk.

Preparation

1. Choose your fish. Not every fish was meant to be fried. The majority of white fish varieties will work well for you if you choose a fish with a more bland flavor and less oil content.

2. Prepare the fish. After giving the fish a thorough rinse, pat dry with paper towels

3. Prepare the breading. Beat one egg and half a cup of milk together in a small bowl. Combine ½ cup bread crumbs, 2 teaspoons roasted onion flakes, 2 teaspoons minced garlic, and 1 teaspoon blackened seasoning in a separate bowl.

4. Cover the fish. Each fillet should be dipped in the egg mixture and then gently pressed into the crumb mixture on both sides.

5. Deep-fry the fish. In a big skillet over medium heat, combine 2 tablespoons butter and 1 ½ teaspoon olive oil. Place the two fillets in the skillets and cook for about three minutes on each side, or until brown.

Pan-fried Poultry

Ingredients

➢ Poultry (like chicken or turkey), Salt, Pepper, Flour, Butter, Olive oil.

Preparation

1. Sprinkle salt and pepper over the chicken.
2. Coat the chicken with flour.
3. In a pan over medium-high heat, stir in the olive oil and butter.
4. Cook the chicken until it turns golden brown on both sides.

RECIPE 10

Cream Sauces and Soups with Low-fat or Fat-free Milk

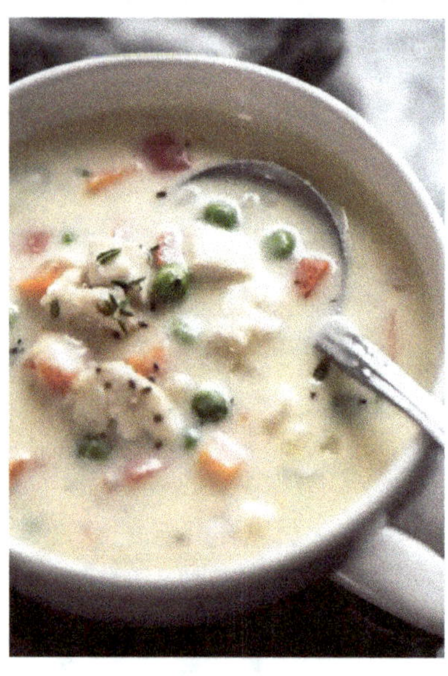

Ingredients

➤ 2 cups of low-fat or nonfat milk, 3 tablespoons cornstarch.

Preparation

1. In a heavy-bottomed saucepan, heat 2 cups low-fat or nonfat milk over medium-low heat.

2. In a small bowl, combine 3 tablespoons cornstarch with 1/4 cup milk.
3. Add cornstarch mixture to the warming milk and stir until smooth.
4. Cook, stirring constantly, for 3 to 4 minutes, making sure the sauce doesn't burn.

RECIPE 11

Roasted Chicken Breast with Lemony Broccoli

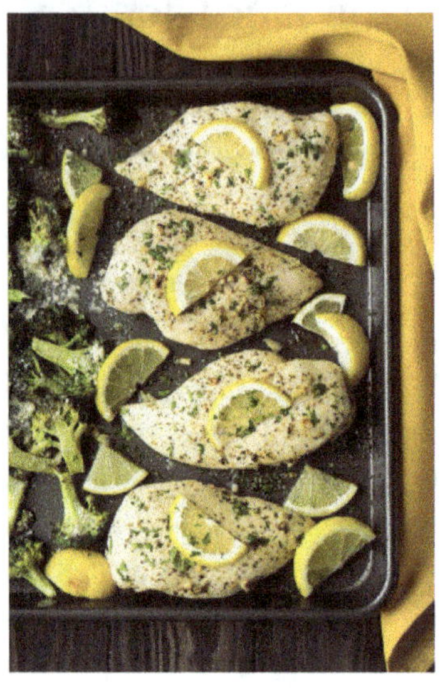

Ingredients

- ➢ 4 (6 oz) boneless, skinless chicken breasts
- ➢ 1 lb broccoli florets
- ➢ 3 Tbsp olive oil
- ➢ 1 Tbsp lemon zest
- ➢ 3 Tbsp fresh lemon juice
- ➢ 3 cloves garlic, minced
- ➢ Salt and freshly ground black pepper
- ➢ 1/2 cup finely shredded parmesan cheese

➢ Chopped fresh parsley and lemon slices for garnish (optional)

Preparation

1. Set oven temperature to 425 degrees Fahrenheit, or 220°C. Put parchment paper on the rim of an 18 by 13-inch baking sheet.
2. To equalize thickness, pound the thicker sections of chicken breasts. Arrange the chicken on one half of the baking sheet and the broccoli florets on the other.
3. Combine olive oil, lemon zest, lemon juice, and garlic in a small mixing basin. Over the chicken and broccoli, evenly drizzle mixture. To taste, add salt and pepper to everything.
4. Roast the chicken breasts in the preheated oven for 16 to 22 minutes, or until the chicken breasts are 165 degrees in the middle and the broccoli is soft and well browned throughout. Take out of the oven, sprinkle the broccoli with Parmesan, and then, if you'd like, sprinkle the chicken with parsley and top

with slices of lemon. Add extra salt to the chicken to suit your taste. Warm servings are recommended.

RECIPE 12

Old-Fashioned Oatmeal

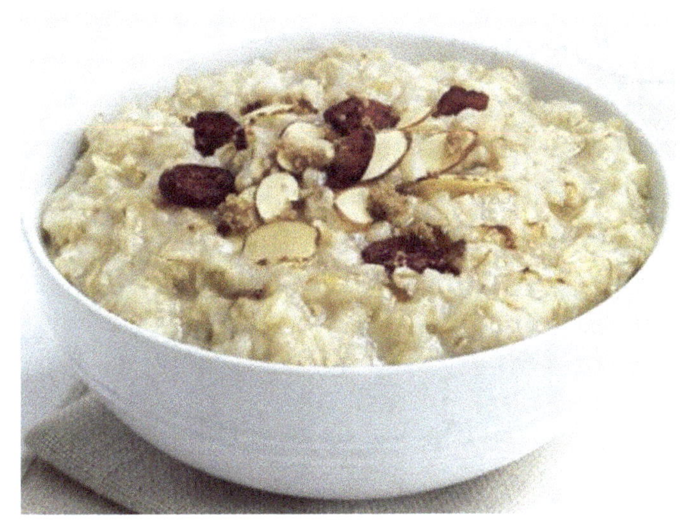

Ingredients

- ➢ 1 cup water
- ➢ 1/2 cup old-fashioned rolled oats
- ➢ 1/8 tsp salt
- ➢ Milk, sweetener, cinnamon, dried fruits or nuts, if desired

Preparation

1. In a small saucepan, mix the milk or water with the salt. Heat up until boiling.
2. After adding the oats, lower the heat to medium and simmer for five minutes, stirring often.
3. After taking off the heat, cover and leave for two to three minutes.
4. If preferred, sprinkle almonds, cinnamon, milk, sweetener, or dried fruit on top.

RECIPE 13
Veggie Hummus

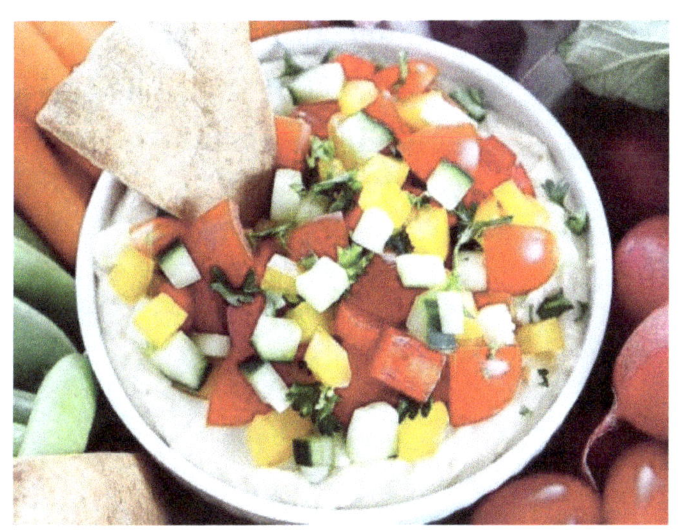

Ingredients

- ➢ 1 container Sabra Classic Hummus
- ➢ 2 tablespoons diced cucumbers
- ➢ 2 tablespoons diced yellow bell pepper
- ➢ 2 tablespoons diced red bell pepper

➤ Chopped parsley for garnish (optional)

Preparation

1. Top the hummus with diced tomatoes, peppers, and cucumbers in a bowl.
2. Add some finely chopped parsley.
3. Accompany with crackers, chips, pita chips, and/or chopped veggies.

RECIPE 14

Turkey Pumpkin Chili

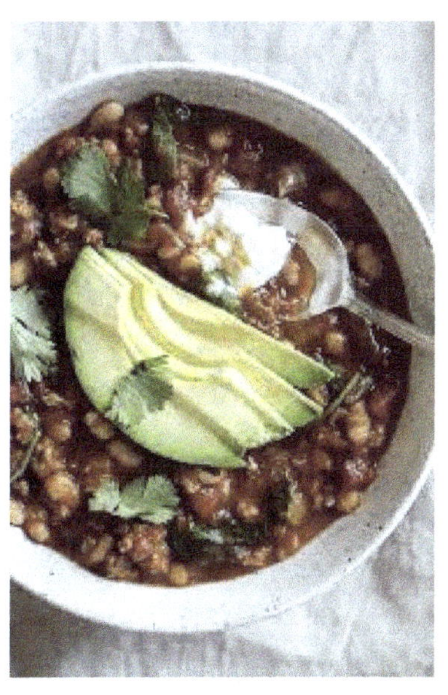

Ingredie nts

- ➢ 1 large yellow onion, diced (about 2 cups)

- ➢ 1 medium bell pepper, red, yellow, or orange, diced

- ➢ 6 garlic cloves, minced (or 3/4 teaspoon garlic powder)

- ➢ 1⅓ pounds ground turkey or chicken, 90 to 93 percent lean

- ➢ One 15-ounce can white beans, drained and rinsed

- ➢ One 28-ounce can diced tomatoes with liquid

- ➢ ¼ cup tomato paste, no salt added
- ➢ One 14-ounce can pumpkin puree
- ➢ 1 cup reduced-sodium chicken or vegetable broth
- ➢ 1 tablespoon chili powder
- ➢ 1 teaspoon ground cumin
- ➢ 1 teaspoon paprika
- ➢ 1/2 teaspoon dried oregano
- ➢ 1/4 teaspoon cayenne pepper (optional)
- ➢ Salt and freshly ground black pepper, to taste
- ➢ For serving: chopped fresh cilantro, diced avocado, diced red onion, plain Greek yogurt, shredded cheese, etc.

Preparation

1. The onion and bell pepper should be cooked for about five minutes over medium heat in a big saucepan or Dutch oven.
2. Cook for 30 seconds after adding the garlic.

3. Include the turkey meat and simmer, breaking it up as it cooks, until it is browned.
4. Add the chili powder, cumin, paprika, oregano, chopped tomatoes, tomato paste, pumpkin puree, broth, salt, black pepper, and cayenne (if using).
5. Increase the heat to a boil, then lower it and simmer for half an hour.
6. You can top with Greek yogurt, cheese, avocado, red onion, cilantro, or whatever else you'd want.

RECIPE 15
Stuffed Pepper Soup

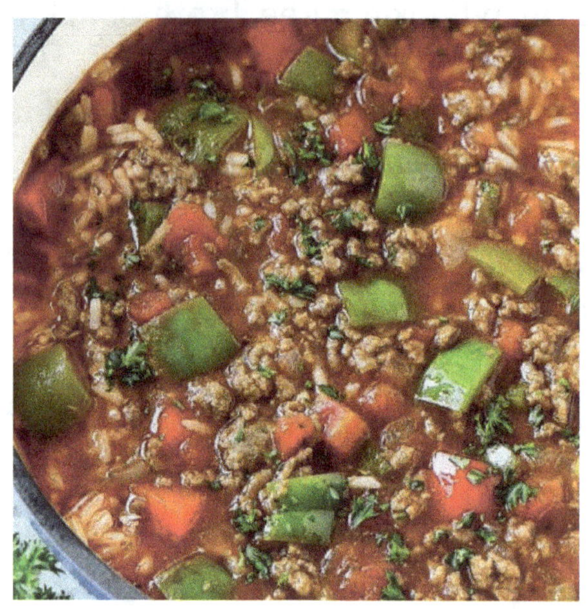

Ingredients

- ➢ 2 tablespoons olive oil
- ➢ 1 large yellow onion, chopped (about 2 cups)
- ➢ 3 cups chopped bell pepper, any color (from 3 bell peppers)

- ➢ 6 garlic cloves, chopped (about 2 tablespoons)
- ➢ 2 teaspoons smoked paprika
- ➢ 1 teaspoon kosher salt
- ➢ 1 teaspoon ground cumin
- ➢ 1 pound lean ground beef (85:15)
- ➢ 1 (15-ounce) can crushed tomatoes
- ➢ 4 cups beef broth
- ➢ 1 (8.8-ounce) package precooked microwavable white rice
- ➢ 6 ounces sharp white Cheddar cheese, shredded (about 1 1/2 cups)
- ➢ Chopped fresh flat-leaf parsley, for serving

Preparation

1. Turn up the heat to medium in a large Dutch oven. When the veggies are soft, about 8 minutes, add the onion, bell pepper, garlic, paprika, salt, and cumin. Stir often.

2. Turn up to medium-high heat and add the ground beef, stirring. For about six

minutes, or until the meat is cooked through, heat while frequently stirring with a wooden spoon to break it up into smaller pieces. Drain out most, but not all, of the fat if there's a lot of it in the pan.

3. Combine the rice, beef broth, and crushed tomatoes. Simmer the soup for about 25 minutes, or until the flavors are well-integrated, after bringing it to a boil over medium-high heat.

Serve garnished with parsley and shredded cheese.

RECIPE 16

White Bean & Sun-Dried Tomato Gnocchi

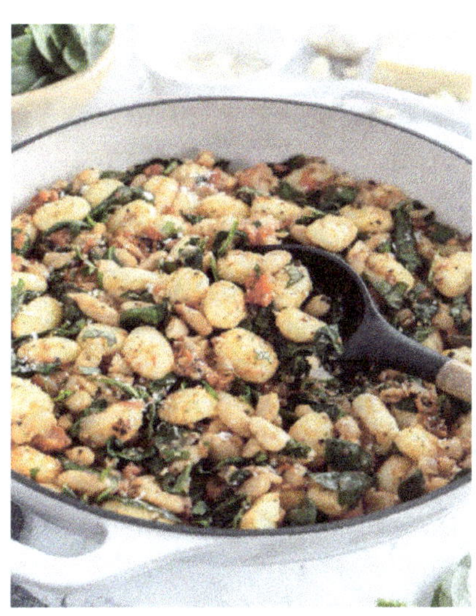

Ingredients

- ➢ 1 package shelf-stable gnocchi
- ➢ 1/2 cup sliced oil-packed sun-dried tomatoes plus 2 tablespoons oil from the jar, divided
- ➢ 1 (15 oz) can low-sodium cannellini beans, rinsed
- ➢ 1 (5 oz) package baby spinach
- ➢ 1 large shallot, minced
- ➢ 1/3 cup low-sodium no-chicken broth or chicken broth

> ➢ 1/3 cup heavy cream

> ➢ 1 tablespoon lemon juice

> ➢ 1/4 teaspoon salt

> ➢ 1/4 teaspoon ground pepper

> ➢ 3 tablespoons fresh basil leaves

Preparation

1. In a large, nonstick skillet, heat up 1 tablespoon of oil over medium-high heat. Add gnocchi and simmer for about 5 minutes, stirring frequently, or until plumped and beginning to brown. Cook the spinach for one minute, or until it has wilted, after adding the beans. Shift over to a platter.

2. Pour in the remaining tablespoon of oil and place the pan over medium heat. Add the shallot and sun-dried tomatoes, and simmer for one minute while stirring. Go to high heat and pour in the broth. Cook for approximately two minutes, or until the liquid has mostly evaporated. After lowering the heat to medium, mix in the cream, lemon juice, salt, and pepper.

3. Add the back to the pan with the gnocchi mixture and swirl to coat in sauce. Sprinkle some basil on top and serve.

RECIPE 17

Chicken & Mushroom Ragu

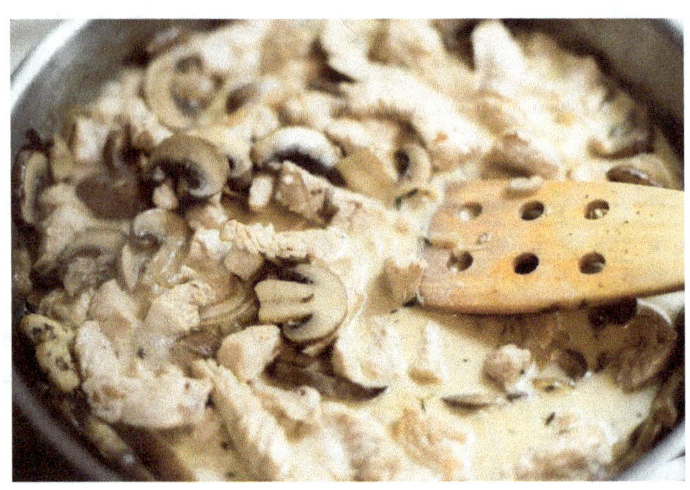

Ingredients

- ➢ 1 medium onion, chopped
- ➢ 2 medium carrots, chopped
- ➢ 8 ounces cremini mushrooms, quartered

- ➤ 1 ¾ pounds boneless, skinless chicken thighs, trimmed and cut into 1-inch pieces
- ➤ 2 cloves garlic, grated
- ➤ ¼ cup tomato paste
- ➤ ½ cup dry red wine
- ➤ ½ teaspoon salt
- ➤ ¼ teaspoon crushed red pepper
- ➤ 1 tablespoon chopped fresh rosemary
- ➤ 1 pound whole-wheat linguine or fettuccine
- ➤ ½ cup grated Romano cheese
- ➤ ½ cup chopped fresh parsley

Preparation

1. Fill a medium-sized bowl with the tomatoes and liquid. Chop the tomatoes into pieces using your palms.
2. To heat oil, use the Sauté mode on an electric pressure cooker. When the mushrooms have shed their juice, which should take around five minutes, add the

onion, carrots, and mushrooms and simmer while stirring.

Add the tomato paste, chicken, and garlic. 3. Simmer for approximately 4 minutes, stirring now and again, or until the chicken is well covered and the bottom mixture starts to turn brown.

4. Include the tomatoes, wine, black pepper, and salt. Sauté for about two minutes, scraping up the browned parts as you go.

5. Cut the heat off. Put the lid away and lock it. Simmer for 10 minutes on high pressure. Turn off the pressure by hand. Stir in the rosemary.

6. In the interim, cook pasta as directed on the package. Remove the excess water and garnish with the cheese, parsley, and sauce.

RECIPE 18

Acorn Squash & Chorizo Tacos

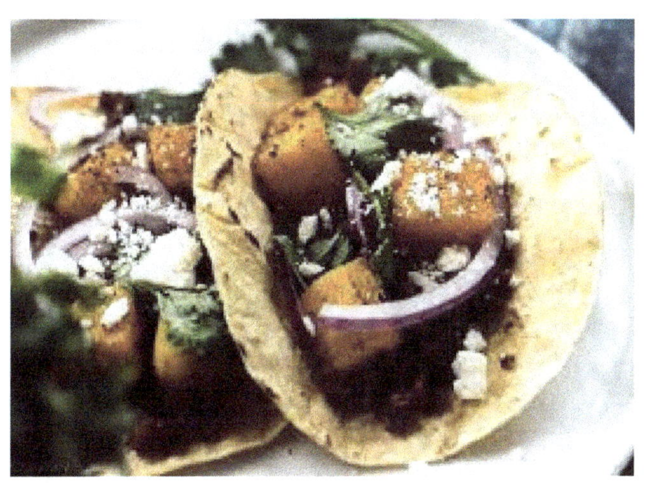

Ingredients

- ➢ 1 medium acorn squash, halved, seeded and cut into 1/2-inch-thick slices
- ➢ 1 medium onion, thinly sliced
- ➢ 2 tablespoons canola oil
- ➢ 1 ½ teaspoons chili powder

- ➢ 1 teaspoon ground cumin
- ➢ ½ teaspoon salt
- ➢ 8 ounces fresh chorizo sausage links (see Tip), halved lengthwise
- ➢ ½ cup sour cream
- ➢ 2 tablespoons lime juice
- ➢ 1 tablespoon chopped fresh cilantro, plus more for garnish
- ➢ 8 corn tortillas, warmed
- ➢ 1 cup shredded red cabbage

Preparation

1. Turn the oven up to 450°F. Combine the squash, onion, oil, cumin, chili powder, and salt in a big bowl. Arrange on a rimmed baking sheet in a single layer. Add some chorizo on top. After stirring halfway through, roast for 20 to 25 minutes, or until the squash is soft and the sausage is thoroughly cooked. 2. Meanwhile, in a separate dish, whisk together sour cream, lime juice, and cilantro.

3. Dice the veggies and chorizo coarsely. Top the tortillas with the crema, spicy sauce, cabbage, and extra cilantro, if preferred.

White Bean Soup with Pasta

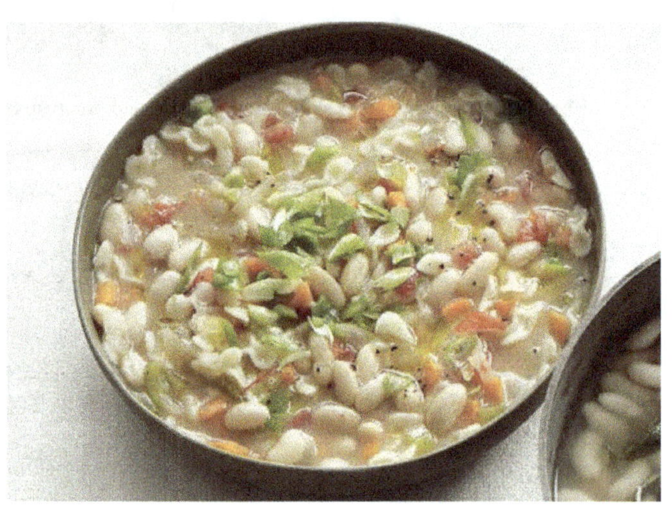

Ingredients

- ➢ 1 tablespoon extra-virgin olive oil
- ➢ 1 ½ cups frozen mirepoix (diced onion, celery, and carrot)
- ➢ 2 cloves garlic, minced
- ➢ 1 teaspoon Italian seasoning

- ➤ 1 teaspoon salt
- ➤ ¼ teaspoon crushed red pepper
- ➤ ¼ teaspoon ground pepper
- ➤ 1 28-ounce can no-salt-added diced tomatoes
- ➤ 2 cups low-sodium no-chicken broth or chicken broth
- ➤ 1 15-ounce can low-sodium cannellini beans, rinsed
- ➤ 8 ounces small whole-wheat pasta, such as elbows
- ➤ 1 ½ cups frozen cut-leaf spinach
- ➤ 4 tablespoons grated Parmesan cheese

Preparation

1. Fill a big saucepan with boiling water.
2. In a large pot over medium-high heat, heat the oil. Add the mirepoix and stir-fry for 3 minutes or until tender.
3. Add the garlic, Italian seasoning, salt, crushed red pepper, and ground pepper. Cook for one minute, stirring occasionally, or until aromatic.

4. Include tomatoes and their juices, beans, and broth; heat to a boil. Lower the heat to keep a vigorous simmer going. Cook with a cover on for around ten minutes, stirring from time to time, or until the tomatoes start to soften.
5. In the meantime, cook the pasta for one minute less than the recipe calls for in the boiling water. Empty the.
6. Blend the soup with spinach. Just before serving, stir in the pasta.
7. Top with a slice of Parmesan.

RECIPE 20

Roasted Honeynut Squash

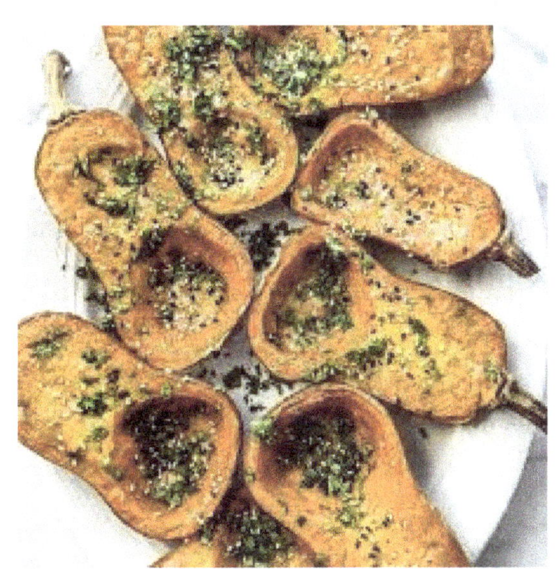

I
n
g
r
e
d
i
ents

- ➤ Honeynut squash
- ➤ Butter
- ➤ Salt
- ➤ Pepper
- ➤ Cinnamon

➢ Maple syrup (optional)

Preparation

1. Get your oven ready for 425°F.
2. Quarter the honeynut squash lengthwise and remove its seeds.
3. Arrange the halves, cut side up, on a baking sheet.
4. Put a teaspoon of butter into each cavity. 5. Season with salt, pepper, and cinnamon. 6. Roast until soft, which should take approximately 25 to 30 minutes.
7. If you like, drizzle with maple syrup.

RECIPE 21
Rainbow Pride Pops

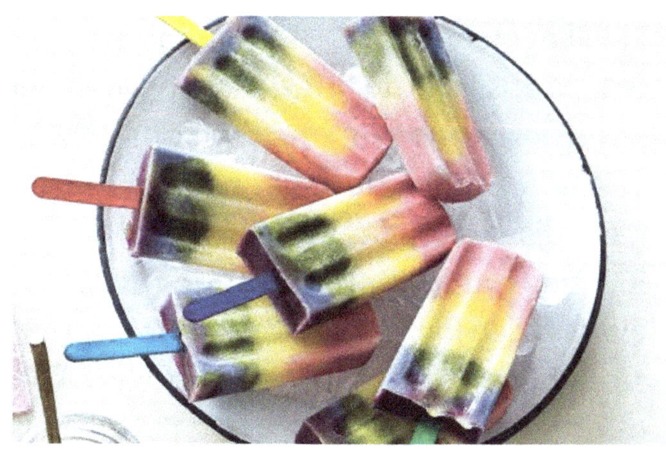

Ingredients

➢ 5 teaspoons each strawberry, orange, lemon, lime, berry blue and grape Jell-O powder

➢ 6 teaspoons superfine sugar

➢ 3 3/4 cups boiling water

Preparation

1. Transfer each flavor of Jell-O to a separate small bowl. Add one teaspoon of superfine sugar to each bowl and whisk.
2. Fill each bowl with 1/2 cup plus 2 teaspoons of hot water, starting with the strawberry and working with one flavor at a time. Once the sugar and gelatin have dissolved, gently stir.
3. Using a tiny liquid measuring cup, evenly distribute 1 tablespoon of the strawberry gelatin (approximately 10 3-ounce ice pop molds) among them. For about 15 minutes, freeze until barely set.
4. Continue with the remaining flavors in the following order: grape, berry blue, orange, lemon, and lime.
5. Insert the wooden sticks into the ice pop mold and replace the cover. Freeze for at least 8 hours or overnight, or until fully solid.
6. Take out of the freezer the pops.

RECIPE 22
Coffee Angel Food Cake

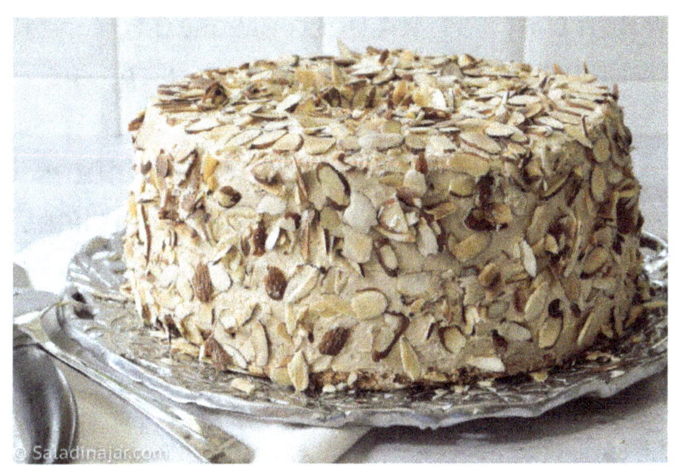

Ingredients

- angel food cake mix
- 1 Tablespoon instant coffee granules
- 1 teaspoon vanilla extract

Preparation

1. Mix the instant coffee and vanilla into the water that the cake mix calls for.

2. Make the angel food cake batter according to the directions on the package. 3. Add the coffee mixture and extracts and mix them in.

3. Pour batter evenly into a 10-inch tube pan that has not been greased.

4. Use a knife to cut through large air pockets in the batter.

5. Bake at 375 degrees for 30 minutes, or until the cake bounces back when lightly touched.

7. Let the cake cool completely before frosting.